The Disability Examination
Your 15th Psychiatric Consultation
William Yee M.D., J.D.
Copyright Applied for 07/19/2020

This missive will start with a broad survey of disability among the mentally ill.

Then I will present my initial psychiatric examination.

The initial examination will have commentary inserted that explains the relevance of each part to the disability examination.

This should allow the medical student, the law student, the health care provider, the patient and other stakeholders understand mental illness and disability.

I will review disability in relation to depression, schizophrenia, and bipolar disorder.

The principles are the same for other forms of mental illness.

Depression will manifest as cognitive deficits in executive function, memory and attention.

The experienced clinician will refer to this as pseudodementia of depression.

Depression will be documented as poverty of thought, psychomotor retardation, anergy, avolition, hopelessness, helplessness to the point of being isolative or even suicidal.

During severe episodes of depression, the patient will not even be able to care for self and may not be safe outside of a psychiatric hospital.

If these depressions are recurrent the patient will be unemployable.

It is estimated that about 30% of patients do not respond to medications.

These patients are not employable.

A substantial portion of depressed patients who respond partially to medications are not employable.

If the depression becomes chronic the patient is unemployable.

Low mood and cognitive impairment cause poor psychosocial functioning that impair all major areas of life activities including employment.

Depression is the second or third cause of disability and affects 5% to 10% of the population.

See:
Collaborative Care for Depression A Cumulative Meta-analysis and Review of Longer-term Outcomes
Simon Gilbody, MBChB, MRCPsych, DPhil; Peter Bower, PhD; Janine Fletcher, MSc; et alDavid Richards, PhD; Alex J. Sutton, PhD
November 27, 2006
Arch Intern Med. 2006;166(21):2314-2321. doi:10.1001/archinte.166.21.2314

"Psychiatric disorders account for 22.8% of the global burden of diseases.[1] The leading cause of this disability is depression, which has substantially increased since 1990, largely driven by population growth and ageing.[2] "

Andrea Cipriani, MD, Prof Toshi A Furukawa, MD, Georgia Salanti, PhD, Anna Chaimani, PhD, Lauren Z Atkinson, MSc, Yusuke Ogawa, MD et al.

The Lancet
VOLUME 391, ISSUE 10128, P1357-1366, APRIL 07, 2018
Open Access Published: February 21, 2018
DOI: https://doi.org/10.1016/S0140-6736(17)32802-7

Depression is a lifelong mental illness.

The depressed patient may present as free of subjective and objective depression during the clinical interview.

The cognitive impairments and disabilities will persist between depressed episodes

Lack of clinical depression does not mean that the impairment has remitted, "94% of patients who had cognitive impairment while depressed continued to experience deficits in cognition when remitted from depression." See:

Cognitive impairment in depression: a
systematic review and meta-analysis
P. L. Rock1, J. P. Roiser, W. J. Riedel, and
A. D. Blackwell
Psychological Medicine (2014), 44, 2029–
2040. © Cambridge University Press 2013
doi:10.1017/S0033291713002535

According to the National Institute of
Health (NIH), schizophrenia affects less
than one percent of the population.

Get the latest research information from
NIH: https://www.nih.gov/coronavirus

Schizophrenia manifests with a disorder
of thought and mood and behavior that is
disabling in all major life activities.

The disorganized thought does not allow
the schizophrenic patient to grasp and
process abstract concepts necessary to
engage in cooperative social transactions.

The disorganized thought results in
disorganized behavior that is disabling in
cooperative activities necessary for the
successful operation of a business.

Disorganized and inappropriate affect impairs social integration necessary for the successful operation of a business.

Hallucinations, delusions, and paranoia all interfere with all major life activities including employment.

Patients with schizophrenia are discharged from military service unfit for service.

Patients with schizophrenia are often discharged from employment on the first day or week of employment due to disruptive or ineffective behavior on the job.

Homelessness is a failure in all major activities of life.

Schizophrenia occurs in approximately 1% of the population. It is present in about 11% of the homeless population. See:
Schizophrenia in homeless persons: a systematic review of the literature
D. Folsom D. V. Jeste

First published: 22 September 2008
https://doi.org/10.1034/j.1600-
0447.2002.02209.xCitations: 83
Dilip V. Jeste Estelle and Edgar Levi
Chair in Aging, Professor of Psychiatry
and Neurosciences, University of
California, San Diego, VA San Diego
Healthcare System, 3350 La Jolla Village
Drive, San Diego, CA 92161, USA E-mail:
djeste@ucsd.edu

Schizophrenia is a chronic mental illness
with generally incomplete remissions and
progressive functional decline during the
lifetime of the patient.
See:
Disability and schizophrenia: a systematic
review of experienced psychosocial
difficulties.
Świtaj, P., Anczewska, M., Chrostek, A. et
al.
BMC Psychiatry 12, 193 (2012).
https://doi.org/10.1186/1471-244X-12-193

Bipolar Disorder affects about 2% of the
population. See:
Prevalence of bipolar disorder in the
general population: a Reappraisal Study

of the Netherlands Mental Health Survey and Incidence Study

E. J. Regeer M. Ten Have M. L. Rosso L. Hakkaart-van Roijen W. Vollebergh W. A. Nolen

First published: 06 September 2004
https://doi.org/10.1111/j.1600-0447.2004.00363.x
Citations: 55

E. J. Regeer, Altrecht GGZ, Lange Nieuwstraat 119, 3512 PC Utrecht, The Netherlands.
E-mail: e.regeer@altrecht.nl

Disability in Bipolar Disorder is due to recurrent episodes and hospital admissions that interfere with a regular work schedule.

Businesses do not function well when employees are absent on an unpredictable basis for uncertain periods of time.

In addition, mood lability and unpredictable behavior is disruptive to productivity and not tolerated by employers.

Even in remission bipolar patients are often low functioning.

During periods of remission bipolar patients suffer from neurocognitive impairment and substantial disabilities in all major life activities including family, social and vocational activities,
See:

Functioning and Disability in Bipolar Disorder: An Extensive Review
Sanchez-Moreno J.a, c · Martinez-Aran A.b · Tabarés-Seisdedos R.d · Torrent C.a · Vieta E.b, e · Ayuso-Mateos J.L.c
Psychother Psychosom 2009;78:285–297
https://doi.org/10.1159/000228249

Another aspect of disability is the period after a psychiatric hospital admission.

One does not expect a patient to go from the hospital to work.

The average length of stay in a psychiatric hospital for depression is six or seven days.

The average length of stay in a psychiatric hospital for schizophrenia is is ten or eleven days.

The average length of stay in a psychiatric hospital for bipolar disorder is seven or eight days.

Average length of stay among mental disorder-related hospitalizations in the U.S. in 2016, by diagnosis
Length of U.S. hospitalizations for mental health in 2016, by diagnosis
Published by John Elflein, Apr 5, 2019
Health & Pharmaceuticals Physicians, Hospitals & Pharmacies

The average length of stay for depression of seven days is much shorter than the average six to eight weeks for an antidepressant medication to work.

This is largely due to the insurance industry using prior authorization to deny continued hospital stay.

The attending physician is required to make a peer to peer call to another psychiatrist to plead for continued hospital treatment.

The peer hired by the insurance industry asks if the patient is in active treatment.

The patient is in the psychiatric hospital with fifteen-minute safety checks.

The psychiatrist is evaluating the patient by informal observation on the unit throughout the day and by at least one formal face to face assessment each day.

The patient is receiving medications administered by nurses daily.

The peer psychiatrist hired by the insurance industry asks the treating psychiatrist if there has been a medication change.

If the treating psychiatrist answers, "no, the patient is still on the single antidepressant," the insurance industry psychiatrist denies continued psychiatric hospital treatment on the premise that, "the patient is not receiving active treatment."

Frequent medication changes are not the best practice in psychiatry.

There is no basis in science to state that a lack of frequent medication changes for a hospitalized patient is lack of active treatment to justify continued payment by the insurance industry.

This is an issue that will eventually support a class action lawsuit against the insurance industry for such short hospital stays for depression in this country.
See:
Released, Relapsed, Hospitalized
Length of Stay and Readmission Rates in State Hospitals a Comparative State Survey,
Doris A. Fuller Chief of Research and Public Affairs Treatment Advocacy Center Elizabeth Sinclair Research Assistant Treatment Advocacy Center John Snook Executive Director Treatment Advocacy Center
Executive Summary
November 2016

In Germany the average length of stay is 36.8 days to 64.3 days.
See:
Duration of inpatient depression treatment--fair benchmarking between hospitals

Multicenter Study Psychother Psychosom
Med Psychol
Mar-Apr 2006;56(3-4):128-37. doi: 10.1055/s-
2005-915331.
[Article in German]
Petra Sitta 1, Silke Brand, Frank
Schneider, Wolfgang Gaebel, Mathias
Berger, Erik Farin, Martin Härter
PMID: 16802418 DOI: 10.1055/s-2005-915331

The literature on the benefits of
antidepressant medication is biased in
favor of benefits.
See:
Selective Publication of Antidepressant
Trials and Its Influence on Apparent
Efficacy
List of authors.
Erick H. Turner, M.D., Annette M.
Matthews, M.D., Eftihia Linardatos, B.S.,
Robert A. Tell, L.C.S.W., and Robert
Rosenthal, Ph.D.
January 17, 2008
N Engl J Med 2008; 358:252-260
DOI: 10.1056/NEJMsa065779

There is research that suggests that the
antidepressant effect is a placebo effect.
See

Listening to Prozac but hearing placebo: A meta-analysis of antidepressant medications.

Kirsch, I., & Sapirstein, G. (1999). Listening to Prozac but hearing placebo: A meta-analysis of antidepressant medications. In I. Kirsch (Ed.), How expectancies shape experience (p. 303–320). American Psychological Association. https://doi.org/10.1037/10332-012

Most experts and treatment algorithms recommend a trial of six to eight weeks for effect before changing the medication See:

Duration of Antidepressant Drug Treatment What Is an Adequate Trial? Frederic M. Quitkin, MD; Judith G. Rabkin, PhD, MPH; Donald Ross, PhD; et alPatrick J. McGrath, MD March 1984 Arch Gen Psychiatry. 1984;41(3):238-245. doi:10.1001/archpsyc.1984.01790140028003

The average length of stay in a psychiatric hospital for schizophrenia is ten or eleven days.
One does not expect a patient to go directly from the hospital to work.

How long should a patient with schizophrenia wait after a hospital admission before attempting to return to work.

That is a clinical decision best made by the treating psychiatrist after several examinations.

There are no simple fool proof tests to determine ability to return to work.

Approximately a third of patients with psychosis have disabilities.
Disability in a Group of Long-stay Patients with Schizophrenia: Experience from a Mental Hospital
Kalita Kamal Narayan and Deuri Sailendra Kumar
Indian J Psychol Med. 2012 Jan-Mar; 34(1): 70–75.
doi: 10.4103/0253-7176.96164
PMCID: PMC3361848
PMID: 22661812

The average length of stay in a psychiatric hospital for bipolar disorder is seven or eight days.

How long should a patient with bipolar disorder wait after a hospital admission before attempting to return to work.

That is a clinical decision best made by the treating psychiatrist after several examinations.

There are no simple fool proof tests to determine ability to return to work.

I have a template for the initial examination of a psychiatric patient that I have been modifying since 1972.

My goal is to do no harm and to help if I can.

To that end the template traps errors.

To that end the template has an audit built in to assure performance improvement.

To that end the template has an introduction to introduce the patient to risks and benefits.

This introduction to risks and benefits allows the patient to have an ability to identify problems as they arise and seek corrective actions to reduce the severity of adverse medication effects.

Review the following and you will have an introduction to the disability examination sufficient to understand what a prima facie case of disability is for Social Security.

"Preexisting text," includes names of symptoms, medical illnesses, medications, people, corporations, law cases, statues, text of statutes, the titles of articles, of books, the content of articles and books cited.
My copyright claim is a clam to the "original text," which is my personal experiences as described in the text above and my commentary on the names of symptoms, medical illnesses, medications, people, corporations, law cases, statues, text of statutes, the titles of articles, of books, the content of articles and books cited.
****

Why I Examine the Patient the Way I Do Error Trapping, Performance Improvement and Auditing
William R. Yee M.D., J.D.

I have been practicing psychiatry without interruption since 1972 in Michigan, Indiana, Kentucky and California.

I have always attempted to do no harm and help if I can according to the Hippocratic Oath and the Golden Rule, treat others as you would have them treat you.

In medical school I was required to take the surgery rotation at Detroit General Hospital in about 1970.

At that time every Friday there was a Morbidity and Mortality Conference.

During that conference all deaths and serious adverse complications of surgery were reviewed by the senior surgeons as an academic exercise in identifying problems and possible strategies for preventing problems from recurring in the future.

The object was not to find fault.

The object was to find a policy, practice and procedure that would trap the error and correct it in the future before it resulted in any repeat of the same error.

The object was to teach the surgeons in training how to function at the same high level as the senior surgeons.

The object was to teach the surgeons in training how to evaluate their own practice and catch errors before they resulted in harm to the patient.

This practice eventually became the basis for Root Cause Analysis taught in most health care facilities.

This practice is a universal practice in all health care organizations that seek accreditation by the Joint Commission. Joint Commission accreditation is often a requirement of health insurance companies for reimbursement for services.

In addition to Friday Morbidity and Mortality rounds, I have been exposed to civil and criminal proceedings in courts.

I have appeared as an expert witness in probate, state, and federal civil and criminal trials in the practice of psychiatry in Michigan, Indiana, Kentucky and California.

I went to law school and was admitted to the Michigan Bar in 1983 to practice law.

My experience as an expert in psychiatry and what I learned in law school made it clear that, "if it wasn't written into the medical record, it didn't happen."

That is why my entries into the medical record tend to be more detailed than entries by my peers.

I am not saying that my practice is better than the practice of other psychiatrists. I am only saying that my notes are more detailed.

Let me summarize the above.

I present myself to the patient as here to do no harm and help if I can.

I have created a template for the first interview to catch errors of omission and correct them before the omission occurs.

I have created a template that includes an audit for written consent for medications, a current AIMS assessment, current and past medications and treatments, known medical conditions, EKG's and labs to monitor medication effects and other important issues in diagnosis and treatment.

There are times when the patient refuses to provide information and consents.

There are times when the patient derails the routine examination so that it cannot be completed during the first visit.

The patient may be depressed and answering so slowly that the next patient arrives before the examination can be completed.

The patient may insist on talking about the narrative they want in the record that does not allow for the complete examination.

We live in an imperfect world and mental illness is an imperfection that provides for a career, employment and an income.

If I do not wish to deal with these inconveniences, I can always find alternative employment.

However, I enjoy the challenge and every "problem" is an opportunity to solve a problem.

I will now examine the initial evaluation through the lens of the Social Security Disability examination.

Before I dissect and explain my initial examination of a psychiatric patient, I will present the following two emails for your consideration:

From: Dr...Redacted
Sent: Wednesday, July 15, 2020 9:28 AM
To: Yee, William

Subject: GA and disability

Hello Dr. Yee,
Hoping to get your insight on disability and general assistance for the AB109 clients. I see that you have seen several of them and they are requesting GA. I'm struggling because I see many of them as capable of working but this has been a disagreement with clinicians.
What are your thoughts when you were working with these clients?
Thanks,
Dr. Redacted

From: Yee, William
Sent: Thursday, July 16, 2020 11:57 AM
To: Dr. Redacted
Cc: Yee, William
Subject: RE: GA and disability

Let us examine the mentally retarded.

Often the mentally retarded have learned to blend in.

They can parrot all the right answers.

But, when you ask them to make a subtle distinction or ask them a question in a different way they become confused.

When you persist, they become distraught.

It is very important to understand what a person can and cannot do.

When you press a mentally retarded patient to do something beyond their capacity, they can become distraught, act out, and require placement into a supervised setting until they can reboot and return to their former level of functioning.

The work environment has become progressively more demanding.

"Productivity," has been assigned as the primary measure for success in the workplace.

This has resulted in EAP's and "burnout," in all industries at all levels.

Composure in a non-stressful environment is the mark of a successful treatment program.

It should not be used as the measure for ability to work.

The history of treatment, the history of being on disability, and the patient's report of ability to function in situations should be given credibility over time.

I understand that people are caught replacing roofs when they are disabled by back injuries.

Replacing one roof is not working eight hours a day week after week.

People endure great hardships out of necessity.

There are malingerers.

There are false positives and false negatives.

As a psychiatrist I do not have a fool proof test.

A judge once told me that an attorney that represents himself has a fool for a client.

My answer was that I have been a fool all my life.

I don't think at the age of 73 with 48 years of experience as a board-certified psychiatrist I can improve upon that answer.

I will give you this information to consider further:
Science & Environment
Most scientists 'can't replicate studies by their peers'
By Tom Feilden
Science correspondent, Today program.

"Science is facing a "reproducibility crisis" where more than two-thirds of researchers have tried and failed to reproduce another scientist's experiments, research suggests.

This is frustrating clinicians and drug developers who want solid foundations of pre-clinical research to build upon.

From his lab at the University of Virginia's Centre for Open Science, immunologist Dr Tim Errington runs The Reproducibility Project, which attempted to repeat the findings reported in five landmark cancer studies.

"The idea here is to take a bunch of experiments and to try and do the exact same thing to see if we can get the same results."

You could be forgiven for thinking that should be easy. Experiments are supposed to be replicable.

The authors should have done it themselves before publication, and all you have to do is read the methods section in the paper and follow the instructions.

Sadly nothing, it seems, could be further from the truth.
After meticulous research involving painstaking attention to detail over several years (the project was launched in 2011), the team was able to confirm only two of the original studies' findings."

If you would like to ask another question, I will do my best to answer.

Thank you for your time and attention. William R. Yee M.D., J.D. Board Certified Psychiatrist.

The Social Security Guidelines are presented here for your considerations: Consultative Examinations: A Guide for Health Professionals
Part III - Consultative Examination Guidelines:
Social Security:
https://www.ssa.gov/disability/professionals/greenbook/ce-guidelines.htm
Claimant's SSN or other non-SSN case identifier and a physical description of the claimant.
Consultative Examination (CE) Report Content
The Consultative Examination (CE) report must:

1. Provide evidence that serves as an adequate basis for disability decision making in terms of the impairment it assesses.

2. Be internally consistent. Are all the diseases, impairments and complaints described in the history adequately assessed and reported in the clinical findings?

3. Do the conclusions correlate the medical history, the clinical examination and laboratory tests, and explain all abnormalities?

4. Be consistent with the other information available within the specialty of the examination requested.

5. Did the report fail to mention an important or relevant complaint within that specialty that is noted in other evidence in the file (e.g., blindness in one eye, amputations, pain, alcoholism, depression)?

6. Be adequate as compared to the standards set out in the course of a medical education.

7. Be properly signed.

My Examination will be presented and dissected and explained as follows:

7/17/2020 face to face started at (commentary: billing is based upon time)

The patient was escorted from the lobby to my office.

The patient made eye contact and extraocular motor movements were intact without evidence of strabismus or nystagmus.

The sclerae were white and without evidence of jaundice.

Station and gait were normal, and patient walked without a cane or walker with a steady gait.

The patient followed a one-step instruction to stand by the door while I wiped down the chair and desk with antiseptic spray.

The patient was maintaining adequate hygiene without a body order, was attentive to grooming, and social conventions.

There were no motor movements indicative of Parkinson's, Tourette's, or Tardive Dyskinesia by informal observation during the time prior to the patient taking the seat in my office. (commentary: appearance and behavior are part of the social security examination and no time with the patient should be wasted because so much information is demanded in a short period of time).

When the patient came into the room the patient was advised that the door was open, and it was the patient's option to leave it open or close it partially or fully for the degree of privacy that the patient wanted.

(commentary: HIPPA requires privacy, but the patient may have more concern about safety and managing anxiety and stress. It is always the patient's choice as to what balance of privacy and stress the patient is willing to accept.)

The patient was advised that leaving the door open reduces the risk of catching COVID-19

(commentary: leaving the door open increases ventilation and dilution of aerosols that accumulate in a room)

The patient was advised if the patient was Claustrophobic or had PTSD from abuse by a male at any time in life it was quite all right to leave the door open.

The patient was advised that if the patient had PTSD and did not feel comfortable in a room alone with a male psychiatrist the patient could have a friend or relative sit in or ask for a female psychiatrist or telepsychiatry.

(commentary: the patient needs to understand that they are free to leave the room any time they want or seek the services of another psychiatrist. It is well known that patients will do better with different psychiatrists of equal competence based upon patient preferences. It is always the patient's choice in these matters.)

I advised the patient that I am here to do no harm and to help if I can.
(commentary: This is the Hippocratic Oath)

The patient was advised that I had practiced since 1972 in Michigan, Indiana, Kentucky and California and had no complaints lodged against me with any licensing board. However, if they wished to lodge a complaint the information was posted and the front office could assist in lodging a complaint
(commentary: California has a requirement that the patient be informed of the right to file a complaint about a medical doctor, and where to file a complaint against a medical doctor. https://www.mbc.ca.gov/Licensees/Notices/Notice_to_Consumers.aspx
Per Business and Professions Code section 138, all California physicians and surgeons are required to inform their patients that they are licensed by the Medical Board of California, and must include the Board's contact information. The information must read as follows:
NOTICE TO CONSUMERS

Medical doctors are licensed and regulated by the Medical Board of California
(800) 633-2322
www.mbc.ca.gov

The purpose of this new requirement (Title 16, California Code of Regulations section 1355.4) is to inform consumers where to go for information or with a complaint about California medical doctors.

Physicians may provide this notice by one of three methods:
Prominently posting a sign in an area of their offices conspicuous to patients, in at least 48-point type in Arial font. (See link "Sign for printing", below, to print the actual notice.

Including the notice in a written statement, signed and dated by the patient or patient's representative, and kept in that patient's file, stating the patient understands the physician is licensed and regulated by the board Including the notice in a statement on letterhead, discharge instructions, or other document given to a patient or the patient's representative, where the notice is placed immediately above the signature line for the patient in at least 14-point type.)

The patient elected to leave the door open during the appointment.
(commentary: I make a record of whether or not the patient closed the door. It is always the patient's choice.)

Are you suicidal or homicidal? "No."
(commentary: I am required to call the police and ask them to take the patient ot a safe place if they are suicidal or homicidal. I work in an outpatient clinic without the resources to keep these patients safe.)

Are you able to drive a car safely? "Yes."
(commentary: I am required to notify the Department of Motor Vehicles if the patient suffers from a medical condition that renders the patient unable to drive safely.)

Chief Complaint, "

(commentary: the patient decides what the patient is willing to treat.)

Current Medications:
(commentary: medications change, and other doctors may be treating the patient and it is important to know all the medications the patient is taking to treat the patient safely.)

Are you having any medication side effects? "No."
(commentary: side effects may require a change in treatment.)

Are you having any physical symptoms such as cough, fever, constipation, diarrhea, nausea, vomiting, rash or other somatic complaints? "No."
(commentary: patients don't always realize that somatic complaints can be side effects that may require a medication change.)

The patient reports problems with teeth as, "none."
The patient is not edentulous.
The patient wears, "no," dentures.

The patient reported motor movement at rest as, "no," none
When asked if the movements disappear when sleeping the patient answered, "I don't know."
The AIMS score today was 0
(commentary: this group of questions addresses the possibility of the side effect of Tardive Dyskinesia. It must be distinguished from Tourette's, Parkinson's, Restless Leg Syndrome and other neurological conditions unrelated to Tardive Dyskinesia.

It is often necessary to advise the patient to have the primary physician authorize a neurology consult or a referral to a sleep clinic for a comprehensive evaluation including a sleep EEG which the psychiatrist does not have access to.

Do you read the package inserts for the medications that you take? "Yes."
(commentary: This addresses the patient's knowledge of medication side effects and the patient's responsibility to participate in the treatment and avoidance of adverse side effects.)

My first psychiatric contact was, "."
I have seen, "." psychiatrists
They have diagnosed me with, "."
They have prescribed the following
medications, "."
I have been in a psychiatric hospital, "."
(commentary: the duration and treatment
of mental illness is necessary to
understand the severity of the mental
illness, the disabling aspects of the mental
illness and the prognosis for recovery and
the ability to work in the future. In
general, the longer the mental illness, the
more hospital admissions, the more
medication trials that have failed, the less
likely that the patient will recover and
return to gainful employment.)

My medical problems include, "."
(commentary: Medical illness contributes
to psychiatric disability and mental
illness contributes to physical disability.
They are synergistic in creating
disabilities of many kinds.)

My allergies are, "."
(commentary: woe to the doctor who
prescribes a medication that the patient is
allergic to.)

My last menstrual period was, "."
(commentary: a fertile woman must be presumed to be pregnant or soon to be pregnant even while on birth control. More than one baby has been born with an IUD in a fist as a trophy of obstacles overcome.)

Gravida "." Para "."
(commentary: these questions bear upon the patient's desire to have more babies and willingness to have an abortion. Birth defects are known risks of any medication.

Fertile women should be encouraged to engage in exercise, meditation, psychotherapy and only accept psychotropic medications if alternative treatments fail and the benefit outweighs the risk.

It is the patient's decision as to whether the benefits outweigh the risks. I have admitted patients to a psychiatric hospital and treated them without medications until after the birth of the child. I was a medical director of a five-county mental health center in Indiana at the time. It was a challenging job, with relatively low pay, and high workload. But, I had powers that I have not enjoyed anywhere else.

Substance Use
Tobacco, "no"
Alcohol, "no"
Street drugs, "no"
I have been in Rehab for drug use or addiction, ""
(commentary: substance abuse impairs treatment, makes mental illness and disability more severe and predicts failure of recovery and return to work.)

I recall my childhood as, "."
(commentary: this often identifies mental illness in childhood. The earlier the onset of mental illness, the more severe the mental illness and the greater the probability of permanent disability.)

When asked if the patient's mother used drugs or alcohol during the pregnancy the patient responded, "no."
(commentary: exposure to drugs and alcohol prior to birth is associated with

brain damage, learning and physical disabilities and permanent disability.)

I was born, "Full Term, Early, Late I don't know what I weighed at birth."
I was born, "Full Term, Early, Late," and weighed, "pounds, ounces."
I, "don't know," if I was full term, early or late."
I was, "healthy," at birth.
I, "don't know," if I was healthy or not at birth.
I had the following medical problems at birth, "."
(commentary: premature birth and health problems at birth are associated with brain damage, learning and physical disabilities and greater frequency of permanent disabilities.)

I, "don't know," when I took my first step, said my first word and other aspects of my childhood development.
I, "did not," attend special education.
I, "did," attend special education, "because
I recall school as, "."
(commentary: The questions above often identify the onset of disabilities prior to

the age of 22, which is a criterion for qualifying for Social Security benefits.)

I completed, "high school in and I have no college."

I completed, "high school in and I have years of college."
(commentary: education is important as a basis for restoring the ability to work.)

I started working when I was, "."
I last worked, "."
"I am not on SSI or SSDI."
"I am on SSI and SSDI."
"I am on Social Security."
(commentary: the history of work and disability is very important for assessing the ability to work and the ability to restoring the ability to work.)

Cultural-Spiritual beliefs and family background,
"I am White,
Native American,
Hispanic, and
Christian,
Baptist,
Pentacostal,

Catholic,
Buddhist."
(commentary: this is important for
identifying resilience and resources for
restoring ability to work or restoring the
ability to live in the community without
supervision.)

Social and relationship History
   I, "have not," been in prison.
   I, "am not," on probation or parole.
   I, "am not," involved in any court cases.
   I am, "straight."

The following people help me when I need
help, "nobody, my spouse, fiance', mother,
father, sisters, brothers, friends.....
   I belong to, "no," church, club or other
social organization.
Do you have a conservator? "No."
Do you have a guardian? "No."
Do you have a payee? "No."
(commentary: this is important for
identifying resilience and resources for
restoring ability to work or restoring the
ability to live in the community without
supervision.)

Abilities I can:

Wash Dishes? "Yes."   "No."
Do Laundry? "Yes."
Take care of children? "Yes."
Cook? "Yes."
House cleaning? "Yes."
 Pay Bills? "Yes."
 Manage Money? "Yes."
Do Taxes? "Yes."
 Keep Doctor Appointments? "Yes."
 Grocery Shop? "Yes."
 Buy clothes? "Yes."
 Find Housing? "Yes."
(commentary: The patient's perception
about ability to live independently is
important in assessing the ability to live
independently in the community.)

My disabilities include, "."
(commentary: The patient's perception
about ability to work or return to work is
important in assessing permanent
disability.)
(commentary: Before starting treatment,
the patient needs to understand the broad
scope of treatments for mental illness.
During the first visit I read the following
to the patient.)

There are many alternative treatments for mental illness that include treatment of medical conditions that cause mental illness.

Some examples are seizure disorders, brain tumors, systemic lupus, and acute intermittent porphyria.

If there is no medical condition causing mental illness, the treatments include aerobic exercise; mental exercise such as meditation; psychotherapies such as CBT, DBT, EMDR or Eye Movement Desensitization and Reprocessing, and many other individual and group therapies which are as effective or more effective than medications for anxiety and depression.

If aerobic exercise; mental exercise such as meditation, and psychotherapies fail, then psychotropic medications should be added to physical exercise, meditation, and psychotherapy.

Before you start psychiatric medications, you should know that about 30% of patients with depression, anxiety, schizophrenia and mental illness in general do not respond to medications.

About 40% of patients with OCD do not respond to medications.

When medications do not work, there are alternatives that require referral from your primary physician to other specialists.

Most insurance policies do not allow the psychiatrist to make the referral.

Alternatives to medications include transcranial magnetic stimulation (TMS) which involves powerful magnets to stimulate the brain; Deep Brain Stimulation involves placing electrodes into the brain for electrical stimulation of the brain; and ECT or electroconvulsive therapy involves electrical shocks to the brain to cause seizures.

Neurosurgery is a final resort when all else fails.

Neurosurgery involves cutting connections in the brain or destroying parts of the brain.

The risks and benefits of these treatments should be discussed with the doctors performing these procedures as they have more knowledge and experience than I do.

Our facility provides psychotherapies and I prescribe medications.

If you choose medications, you need to understand that you can have an allergic reaction to any medication that can be life threatening and may require a visit to the emergency room for immediate treatment.

There may be sudden severe difficulty breathing, sudden severe skin rashes, sudden severe damage to different organs in the body that can be immediately life threatening.

However, psychotropic medications are less likely to cause allergic reactions than penicillin and other antibiotics, except perhaps for lamotrigine.

I have been prescribing psychiatric medications since 1972 and only three patients reported allergic reactions to me.

The rashes resolved when the medications stopped, and the patients took Benadryl.

None of my patients suffered death or permanent injury from allergic reactions.

Some psychotropic medications may case sudden life-threatening heart rhythm abnormalities that can be lethal.

You have the choice of waiting for an EKG before starting psychotropic medications or you can start the medications first and get an EKG second.

I have not had any patient die from these side effects.

There can be severe life-threatening side effects such as neuroleptic malignant syndrome and serotonin syndrome with fast heart rate, high blood pressure, high temperature, muscle damage, kidney failure, coma and death.

However, these are not likely to happen with a low starting dose.

I have not had any patients die or suffer permanent injury from the medications I prescribed, except one elderly lady who had pneumonia in a nursing home, became dehydrated and died from lithium toxicity.

That death could have been avoided if the patient had stopped the lithium with the onset of the pneumonia.

However, the pneumonia was not discovered until after she became dehydrated.

Older people often get silent or asymptomatic pneumonias without a fever. They sleep and do not appear to be in distress.

There are many delayed side effects such as Tardive Dyskinesia, abnormal motor movements at rest; and elevated prolactin levels that cause the breasts of both men and women to enlarge and leak milk.

There are many anticholinergic medications. Many medications for psychosis, depression, anxiety, insomnia, nausea, pain, diarrhea, seizures and other medical problems may cause dry mouth, constipation, blurred vision, drowsiness, falls, memory problems, confusion and hallucinations.

Long term exposure to anticholinergic medications has been found to increase the risk of dementia.

Read the package inserts and discuss the delayed side effects with follow up appointments.

You will not be able to decide regarding taking the medication long term until after you start it, and find out how much it improves your mental health.

Then you can decide if the benefit is large enough to justify the risk of long-term side effects described in the package inserts that you are given with the medications.

Fifty to seventy five percent of patients do not continue psychotropic medications because they do not find the benefit to be worth the cost in time, money and side effects that come with the benefits.

Do you understand? "Yes."

Do you want to ask any questions? "No."

What do you want to do now?
(commentary: After ascertaining the fact that the patient understands the treatments available, it is always the patient's choice as to how to proceed.)

The patient signed consent for,
(commentary: I obtain written consent for treatment with medications.)

The patient gave permission to order and EKG and lab tests.

The following labs were ordered...
The patient was advised to make an appointment in the front office on the way out for a medication renewal before his medications ran out

The patient was advised that he could make PRN appointments for medication adjustments if he had medication side effects or problems with symptoms.

I will offer medication tapers with each appointment.

You may request medication increases or changes at each visit.

The patient reported that he had no more questions.

The patient reported satisfaction with treatment.
(commentary: I educate the patient as to: The need to make appointments before medication reviews leaving the office. The fact that I offer medication tapers to reduce exposure to side effects. The fact that the patient may ask for a medication increase or change if they find the benefit to be greater than the risk.)
face to face ended at
Charting for the Initial Assessment and Medical Progress started at * and finished at *.

(commentary: I document time for billing purposes. I find that many facilities schedule too many patients to provide good care and documentation.)

"Preexisting text," includes names of symptoms, medical illnesses, medications, people, corporations, law cases, statutes, text of statutes, the titles of articles, of books, the content of articles and books cited.

My copyright claim is a clam to the "original text," which is my personal experiences as described in the text above and my commentary on the names of symptoms, medical illnesses, medications, people, corporations, law cases, statues, text of statutes, the titles of articles, of books, the content of articles and books cited.

www.ingramcontent.com/pod-product-compliance
Lightning Source LLC
Chambersburg PA
CBHW021928170526
45157CB00005B/2224